Advance Praise

"In Volume 1 of what will undoubtedly be an essential study on the understanding and effects of ADHD on children, Dr. Dawn Brown systematically and methodically addresses the reality of exercise, nutrition, and a balanced diet for success in the lives of children who sometimes struggle with focused attention despite their scholastic prowess. Her personal stories of championing ADHD in her own life, coupled with her stellar scholarship in this discipline, make this study even more fundamental for every family who has found their child(ren) distracted or daydreaming more often than they would like. I personally appreciate her commitment to balanced diet and proper eating to ensure our brain health and development. Although her message is primarily for children, every age group would do well to take heed to the revelations made in *The ADHD Lifestyle Series, Volume 1*."

—Rev. Dr. Marcus D. Cosby,
Senior Pastor of Wheeler Avenue Baptist Church

"Dr. Brown provides tangible and evidence-informed information for parents whose children experience the challenges of living well with attentional problems. Treatment for attentional disorders can be confusing to parents wishing to do more than have medications prescribed. In this book, she outlines a variety of important lifestyle guidelines that will serve the entire family."

—Laurel L. Williams, DO,
Associate Professor at Baylor College of Medicine

"*The ADHD Lifestyle Series, Volume 1* takes us on an informative journey of learning how to manage symptoms of ADHD. The knowledge that Dr. Brown imparts helps to empower parents to augment pharmacological treatment with a toolbox of healthy nutritional and behavioral strategies for their children. Her transparency of her own experiences with ADHD normalizes and destigmatizes the illness and helps to remind us all that a diagnosis of ADHD does not have to limit a child's success."

—Valdesha Dejuan, MD,
Psychiatrist Pacific Medical Centers

"*The ADHD Lifestyle Series, Volume 1* is an ideal resource for educators, mental healthcare professionals, and parents of children with ADHD. Dr. Dawn Brown does an excellent job of using her own experiences to help readers better understand the role good health and nutrition play in managing ADHD. The strategies and ideas to increase children's fruit and vegetable intake and the tips provided on how to switch out unhealthy snacks with healthier alternatives are helpful and practical. This book is empowering and offers a holistic approach to a better quality of life for those living with ADHD."

—Rockell Brown, PhD,
Assistant Professor at Texas Southern University

The ADHD
Lifestyle Series, Volume 1
Secrets From An MD with ADHD

The ADHD
Lifestyle Series, Volume 1
Secrets From An MD with ADHD

Building Balanced Meals and
Exercise Routines for Children

Dawn Kamilah Brown, MD

purposely
created
PUBLISHING

THE ADHD LIFESTYLE SERIES, VOLUME 1
Published by Purposely Created Publishing Group™
Copyright © 2018 Dawn Brown

Printed in the United States of America
ISBN: 978-1-948400-00-8

Dr. Dawn Psych MD's books and products are available through online book retailers.
To contact DrDawnPsychMD.com directly, call our Customer Service Department within the U.S. at 281-419-ADHD (2343).

Dedication

Thank you, God, for gifting me with a condition that has challenged me, strengthened me, and taught me how to be the best me. Now, I can help others discover that what the world calls a disability is actually their AMAZE-ability!

In honor of my guardian angel, Dr. Sandra Faye Urquhart Brown, PhD, who was my #SuperMom, my confidant, my best friend, and unknowingly to her—my ADHD coach. I am blessed and thankful for the twenty-eight years the Lord allowed us to share. You are truly missed. "To be absent from the body is to be present with the Lord" (2 Corinthians 5:1).

To my dad, Donald Ray Brown, my guide, my protector, my hero. I admire your strength, courage, leadership, and unwavering faith in God. I am grateful for your daily prayers and speaking words of wisdom and Scriptures into my life. You are truly a wonderful man of God.

To my brother, Dr. Donald Rashad Brown II, MD, Forensic Psychiatrist! I cannot express the joy as well as the laughter you bring to my life! Although I may be the older sibling, you are my inspiration and I am proud of the man you have become. I am honored to be your sister.

To ALL my #FocusBuilders #SuperMoms #ADHD-Champs #AllStars:

Thank you for following me on all social media avenues @DrDawnPsychMD and for supporting my products (The ADHD Lunch Box, The ADHD Backpack, and The ADHD Wristminders by Dr. Dawn Psych MD) found on my website, www.DrDawnPsychMD.com. Guess what?! I dedicate this book to all of you!

Some people believe it, but living with ADHD is not a hardship or battle. It's actually a creative experience where you learn to build structure, routines, and confidence that leads to success!

Volume one begins the journey to live optimally with *Building Balanced Meals and Exercise Routines for Children.* This volume will provide you with foods, nutrients, vitamins, and minerals that are beneficial for ADHD minds, and includes a few recipes and tips to assist you with making those awesome meals that will positively impact your child's behaviors. It also includes recommended age-appropriate mind and physical exercises that can help increase your child's attention span, energy levels, and impulse control.

Before you read *The ADHD Lifestyle Series, Volume 2: Secrets from an MD with ADHD: Building Organizational Tools and Simple Home Routines to Champion Your Child's ADHD* and *The ADHD Lifestyle Series, Volume 3: Secrets from an MD with ADHD: Building Classroom Strategies and Brain Health Activities to Empower Your ADHD Child*, it is important to first recognize the essential fuel and fun activities that our

ADHD brain needs to function optimally. This volume also addresses the supplemental product, The ADHD Lunch Box, which is a cool invention to motivate your child to pack their own lunch. It also includes healthy meal options that will assist with their educational achievements.

So, what are you waiting for?! Enjoy reading and learning from a book that was written for YOU by a doctor that proudly lives with and has championed her ADHD!

Table of Contents

Introduction

I realized that creating a healthy diet and exercise routine were key factors to help manage my ADHD symptoms. My focus didn't improve until my meals contained the essential vitamins, minerals, nutrients, and foods that the brain uses as fuel to do its job effectively. Once I changed my diet, my focus duration increased, my memory improved, my motivation heightened, and my energy levels sustained. These factors led to me being a successful doctor, keen listener, avid learner, better communicator, and an ultimate achiever at home, work, and in my social life! I wasn't aware that certain foods are disguised as being healthy although they contain harmful ingredients that do not promote brain health, particularly for executive functioning (learning, processing, understanding, planning, organizing, and behaving).

After I found success with making dietary changes in my life, my next thought was to share those changes with the world! Within this book lies the answers to how I achieved a balanced diet and discovered behaviors that helped me to champion my ADHD.

This volume of *The ADHD Lifestyle Series* will help parents build healthy diets and exercise routines for kids of different ages who have ADHD.

1. It will provide the building blocks to help establish healthy eating habits that they can begin TODAY for the best start in life. What kids eat now impacts their ADHD symptoms, health, behaviors, fitness, and what they will eat in the future.

2. It will provide tips to create and maintain a healthy meal plan by giving suggestions on how to involve kids with ADHD in meal preparation, shopping, and cooking activities. When you read these chapters, remember three key recommendations: 1- Don't ban food (this increases kids urges), 2- Don't use food for rewards, 3- Encourage your kids to eat in moderation.

3. It will promote actual results. Let's face it. It can be difficult to change our diet, so just imagine trying to change your child's. Here is a free tip: Be REAListic when encouraging healthy dieting for your children. Exercise the 80/20 rule—encourage a balanced diet 80 percent of the time and allow your kiddos to enjoy foods they want 20 percent of the time.

4. It will provide tips on how to be successful by helping YOU first. Did you know that if a parent has ADHD, a child has more than a 50 percent chance of having it? That's right!! Your odds of having ADHD are 50/50. With this fact in mind, it is important that you BE an EXAMPLE. Start early with your

kids (meal plans will be suggested for different age groups). Be consistent (establish a routine). Be persistent (taste buds change). Establish meal times (sit at the dinner table). Balance their diet with exercise (i.e., age-appropriate sports).

You see? This is the book that you have been waiting for! Better yet, it is followed by additional volumes that address equally important management tools to help you and your ADHD child succeed! From my personal experience living with ADHD, I am delighted to show you how to help active minds (ADHD kids) achieve by creating routines for eating a balanced meal and participating in age-appropriate activities and exercises. Let's get started!

CHAPTER 1

What Is ADHD?
Could My Child Have It?

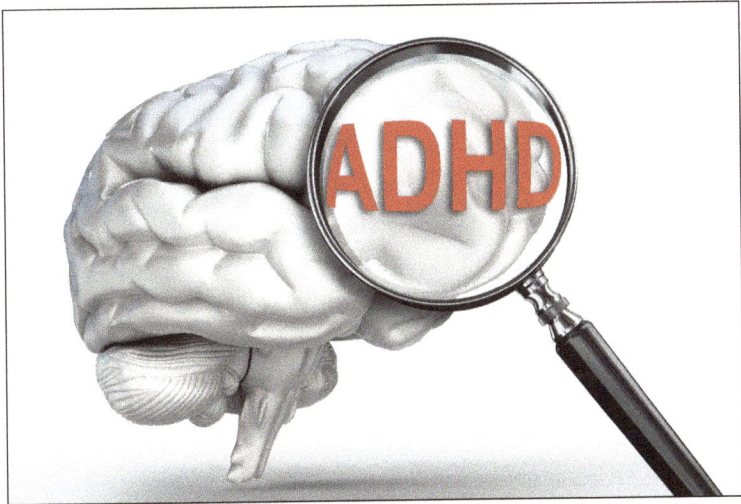

I was an honor roll student but not without challenges. I was also known to be a "social butterfly." The comments on my report cards stated, "Excellent student. Well-liked by all her peers. Puts in a lot of effort. Makes careless mistakes. Requires more time for some assignments. Very sociable." When my parents discussed the teachers' comments with me, I thought most were not a problem since I made good grades. However, it was discovered that when I appeared bored in class and finished work early, I became distracted and talked to my peers. Thus, the "social butterfly" emerged.

My mother made me read books after I read my first word and picked out all of my teachers throughout elementary school. I studied for hours and worked with my dad, who is known as a "math whiz." In class, I recall having to re-read passages in books because I often daydreamed. I would ask my classmates to repeat what the teacher taught out of fear of being told I was not a good listener. I was afraid of my name being placed on the board because I knew that I would get into trouble at home. I was also known to many as a teacher's pet, partly because my peers often witnessed them encouraging me. Later, I would understand that many of the symptoms I displayed throughout my education were apart of ADHD. I was not diagnosed with ADHD until age 32.

WHAT IS ADHD?

Attention-Deficit/Hyperactivity Disorder, also known as ADHD, is a common childhood mental health disorder and can continue into adulthood. There are three subtypes of ADHD: Predominantly Inattentive (formerly known as ADD), Hyperactive-Impulsive, and Combined (Hyperactive-Impulsive and Inattentive). Kids with ADHD have difficulties with paying attention and staying focused. They struggle with trying to control their behaviors, and they may appear to be hyperactive (over-active). A combination of factors can cause ADHD. In addition to genetics, researchers are studying how brain injuries, in utero exposure to smoking, nutrition, and environmental factors might contribute to ADHD.

COULD MY CHILD HAVE ADHD?

Children are naturally full of energy, highly talkative, and impulsive. It is typical for a child to require reminders for completing a task, need assistance with locating a toy they misplaced, and encounter challenges with sitting still at the dinner table. ADHD is the most common mental health disorder in children, but it does not mean the majority of kids have it. One way to know if your child has ADHD is through a series of evaluations with a mental health professional. Although they may have some symptoms that seem like ADHD, it might be something else.

HOW IS ADHD DIAGNOSED?

Diagnosing ADHD is a process that may involve several steps of your child's doctor gathering information from multiple sources. Doctors should use standard guidelines developed by the American Academy of Pediatrics.

A physician will complete a comprehensive medical history and a physical exam. They will ask details about your child's symptoms, how long the symptoms have occurred, and how the behavior affects your child, their friendships, and the rest of your family.

ARE THERE TESTS USED TO DIAGNOSE ADHD?

There is no definitive test for ADHD. However, behavior rating scales for ADHD can help measure and compare your child's behavior with their peers. These tests contain scales that evaluate inattention, hyperactivity, and impulsivity to determine the ADHD type. Kids, caregivers, and teachers should be involved in this process.

Doctors may request that your child complete lab work to evaluate for other medical conditions that are known to cause symptoms like ADHD. Some doctors may even suggest ordering a noninvasive brain scan.

A doctor's comprehensive evaluation, the use of behavior rating scales, and a child's interview are equally important to help determine a diagnosis.

HOW YOUNG IS ADHD DIAGNOSED?

I have evaluated children for ADHD as young as preschool age. Children in this age group usually come to my office when they are challenged with severe and frequent behavior concerns. However, diagnosing ADHD in children younger than five can be difficult because many preschool children naturally have some of the symptoms seen in ADHD. Also, a child's behavior and development change very rapidly during the preschool years.

How is ADHD Diagnosed?	Key facts about Diagnosing ADHD
Commonly seen in children ages four to eighteen. Child shows six or more specific symptoms of inattention or hyperactivity or impulsivity. Symptoms must begin by age twelve. Symptoms are consistent. Symptoms must occur for more than six months in at least two settings. Doctor compares child's behavior with that of other children the same age.	**HOW DOES ADHD AFFECT A CHILD'S LIFE?** Children with ADHD have major problems in one or more areas of their life, such as their school performance, friendships, and relationships with family. **WHERE DO THE SYMPTOMS APPEAR?** Symptoms must be present in at least two settings, such as at home and school. They also show up in social scenes (i.e., Boy Scouts, dance class).

CHAPTER 2

Strategies for Managing ADHD

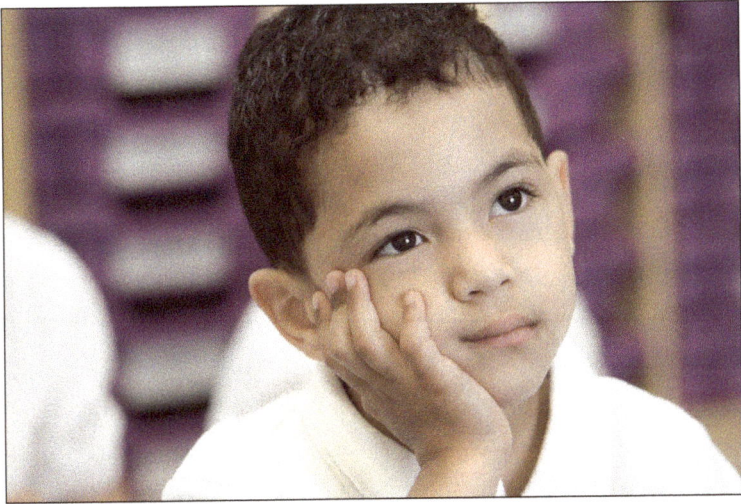

After being diagnosed with ADHD and advised on the treatment methods, I was initially resistant. I did not want to take medication or follow any of the treatment plans. I had to come to terms that this was a disorder that required daily management in order for me to function optimally and be successful in life.

Once your child is diagnosed with ADHD, an individualized treatment plan based on the best available science and management options for your child is discussed. There is an art to ADHD management. There is not just one method that manages ADHD optimally.

1. Medication Therapy

   Research shows that medication therapy is the most effective management for most children. 80 percent of the kids who take medications perform optimally if the type and dosage are at the right therapeutic level.

   There are two main kinds of medication for ADHD: stimulants and non-stimulants. They work differently in the brain to help control ADHD symptoms. These medications can have side effects that usually go away a few days after starting treatment. If not, the prescriber may suggest trying a different dose to see if that will work better, or they may recommend changing the medication. It is equally important to evaluate for other common reasons why a child may experience side effects. For example, insomnia due to taking their medication too late or stomachaches because of their failures to eat a well-balanced meal.

   There are also alternative medications available over-the-counter (OTC) that aren't recognized by the FDA as treatment options. These are called supplements and it is important to know that the law does not regulate them.

Experiencing anxiety and depressive symptoms are common for kids with ADHD. For these kids, doctors may recommend additional medication or therapy.

2. Behavior Management

Therapies may help kids manage their ADHD symptoms. Some do best with a combination of treatments. These therapies occur with a mental health provider.

a. ADHD Coaching- Provides strategies to help children with ADHD and their families succeed. The goal is to improve their day-to-day living by teaching an organized approach to learning and completing tasks. Strategies to help kids with motivation are also used.

b. Behavioral Therapy- Changes negative behaviors into positive ones, while supporting positive behaviors.

c. Cognitive Behavioral Therapy (CBT)- Focuses on children talking about their thoughts, feelings, and behaviors.

d. Parent Management Training- Provides caregivers with practical solutions for the social, emotional, and behavioral challenges they experience with their children.

e. <u>Individual and Family Therapy</u>- Provides children and their caregivers with additional opportunities to understand ADHD. They learn ways to develop and nurture the necessary skills to manage symptoms, help improve family relationships, and support their overall success.

f. <u>Social Skills Groups</u>- Helps kids learn and practice fundamental skills for interacting with others.

3. Food and Nutritional Meal Planning

Nutritional meal planning has been used by many as an alternative treatment for ADHD. Now, it is more commonly a part of the combined treatment plan along with other treatment options. Nutritional meal planning for ADHD management focuses on eliminating certain foods, adding dietary supplements, choosing healthy foods to help reduce ADHD symptoms, or a mixture of the three.

4. ADHD and Sleep Problems

Children who have ADHD and children who have sleep problems may have similar signs such as hyperactivity, inattentiveness, and restlessness. One might be mistaken for the other because of the overlap of symptoms. The majority of kids with ADHD struggle more with going to sleep versus staying asleep. It is important for their bedtime routine to promote sleep, which includes turning off all electronics (video games, tablets, TV), taking a bath, and reading a bedtime story.

I never liked going to bed on time. Till this day, I must "make myself" go to bed. I am very energetic at night, and I believe it is the time when my thoughts are most creative. As I age, I realize that sleep is very important for my brain and body. My brain needs to sleep too, especially after being very active with thoughts throughout the day. I also learned that when I did not get enough sleep, I became moody, tired, and fatigued. I struggled with being motivated to accomplish tasks and felt less energetic, particularly during the early evenings. I became more distracted and my thoughts weren't as sharp. After I worked on my sleep hygiene routine, all of these areas improved. I noticed I felt great, performed optimally, and produced my best work.

5. Exercise Therapy

In general, exercise helps children function better and feel better. Research shows that regular physical activity decreases the severity of ADHD symptoms and improves cognitive functioning in children.

ADHD AND SLEEP PROBLEMS

ADHD may relate to trouble sleeping in the following ways:

1. Having unmanaged ADHD is the reason why problems with sleep result.

2. Sleep difficulties are related to other disorders that co-occur with ADHD (i.e., anxiety).

3. The late timing of a stimulant medication prevents good sleep hygiene.

4. No relation with ADHD (sleep problems are just common in general).

5. It is estimated that at least 25 percent of all children, not just those with ADHD, will develop a sleep disorder in their lifetime. Poor sleep has varying impacts on family dynamics, school achievement, and other health issues. You should talk to your doctor if you are concerned about your child's sleep hygiene.

CHAPTER 3

A Few Myths About Food's Impact on ADHD

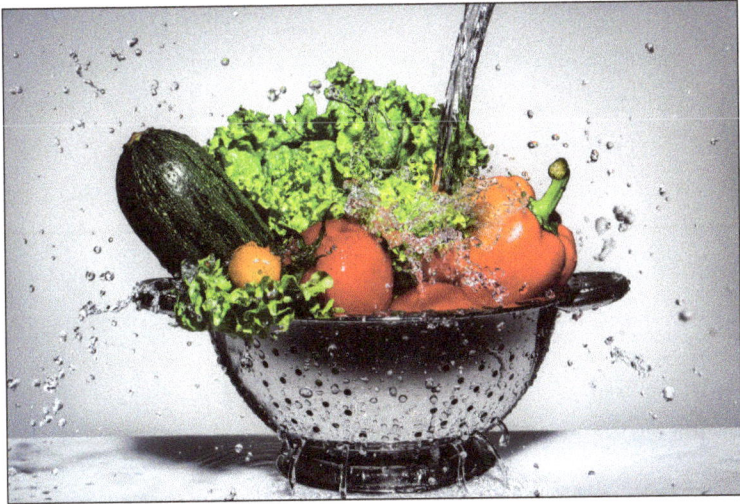

Myths regarding food and ADHD have developed over the years. Let's debunk these myths with facts:

SUGAR

<u>Myth</u>: Sugar causes hyperactivity and can make ADHD symptoms worse.

<u>Fact</u>: Studies have examined this idea and found that sugar does not cause ADHD symptoms. Several studies have concluded that sugar may cause periods of hyperactivity in children, followed by sedation and inactivity. It also impacts other aspects of health such as bloating and inflammation, weight gain, cavities, and other health insensitivities unrelated to ADHD.

I now realize that sugar is in almost every food product we consume. It's one ingredient that is hard to not eat and can be rather addictive. I crave the three c's: cakes, cookies, and chocolate! When I reached my 20's, I noticed that when I included less sugar in my meal plans, I actually lost weight and felt great! Although sugar is an ingredient that I still crave, I am more conscientious of how it impacts my thoughts, moods, weight, and optimal functioning.

GLUTEN

<u>Myth</u>: Gluten-enriched foods can cause ADHD symptoms.

<u>Fact</u>: For many years, gluten-free diets have been suggested for ADHD symptoms. Studies in 2011 concluded that individuals with both Celiac disease and ADHD saw an improvement in their ADHD symptoms, following treatment

for Celiac disease. However, gluten-free diets did not have an impact on ADHD symptoms if the child did not have Celiac disease. There is no known direct association with Celiac disease and ADHD although both conditions have associated food allergies.

VITAMIN OR TRACE MINERAL DEFICIENCY

Myth: Multivitamins can cure ADHD symptoms.

Fact: Unfortunately, resolving ADHD symptoms is not as simple as adding a multivitamin, although studies have shown those with ADHD to be deficient in certain vitamins and minerals. However, this deficiency is not found to cause ADHD, nor does replacing vitamins and minerals help with symptom control.

ARTIFICIAL COLORS OR PRESERVATIVES

Myth: Artificial colors or preservatives found in food can cause ADHD.

Fact: Studies have not concluded that artificial colors or preservatives cause ADHD. However, some children and adults (regardless of an ADHD diagnosis) have sensitivities to artificial colors and preservatives. Increased activity and focus difficulties have been observed.

ORGANIC VS. CONVENTIONAL FOODS

Myth: There is a direct link to pesticides and ADHD.

Fact: Preliminary research suggests that pesticides might play a role in causing ADHD, but a certain relationship has not been confirmed. Using a veggie wash and choosing organic foods helps reduce pesticide exposure for children and expectant moms.

FOOD ALLERGIES VS. FOOD SENSITIVITIES

Myth: Food allergies and sensitivities can cause ADHD.

Fact: When food causes an allergic reaction, serious symptoms of swelling, hives, and anaphylaxis can occur. This is a different reaction from food sensitivities, which produce symptoms such as hyperactivity and inattention and can be mistaken for ADHD. A referral to an allergist is recommended if a food allergy is suspected.

PESTICIDES

Myth: Decreasing pesticide exposure will improve ADHD symptoms in children (or adults) *who already have ADHD*.

Fact: Evidence suggests that high pesticide exposure *doubles* the risk of a child acquiring ADHD. However, the alternative (decreasing exposure) is not true.

CHAPTER 4

Overall Nutrition – "It's Not a Diet, It's a Lifestyle"

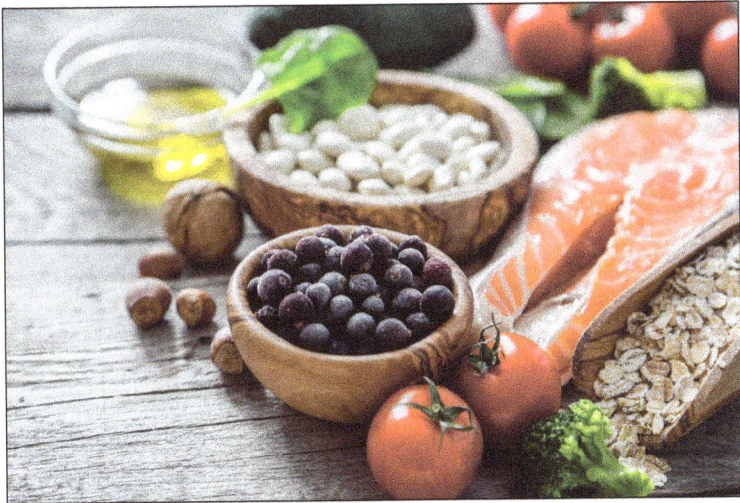

Nutritional meal plans used in place of traditional ADHD treatments have proved "unsatisfactory or unacceptable" (The Journal of Pediatrics, January 2013). Clinical observations suggest that meals rich in fiber, folate, and omega-3 fatty acids help reduce hyperactivity and positively impact cognitive development and performance. These components alone will not treat ADHD symptoms but will increase the likelihood of achieving good health.

REMEMBER THE THREE F'S

1. Omega-3 **Fatty Acids**

   Fatty acids are essential components for cognitive development, protecting the heart, strengthening the immune system, providing body insulation, and maintaining a healthy metabolism and weight.

2. **Fiber**

   Fiber is crucial for maintaining proper digestive health. It helps relieve and prevent constipation.

3. **Folate**

   Folate is a natural B9 vitamin. It is important for cell growth and in the formation of DNA. Low levels of folate are associated with an increased risk of the following health conditions: heart disease and stroke, cancer, and birth abnormalities of the nervous system.

Foods listed below are high in these vital nutrients. Consider adding them to your family's diet lifestyle!

FOODS HIGH IN OMEGA-3 FATTY ACIDS

- ❯ Fish: mackerel and salmon
- ❯ Oils: olive, coconut, flaxseed, and sesame
- ❯ Organic, grass-fed beef
- ❯ Vegetables: collard greens, broccoli, and spinach
- ❯ Avocados
- ❯ Walnuts
- ❯ Sesame and flax seeds

FOODS HIGH IN FOLATE

- ❯ Asparagus
- ❯ Beans
- ❯ Soybeans
- ❯ Dried herbs
- ❯ Sunflower seeds
- ❯ Dark green, leafy vegetables like collard greens, broccoli, and spinach

FOODS HIGH IN FIBER

- Whole grains
- Beans
- Fruit
- Vegetables

OVERALL NUTRITION CONSISTS OF THESE "MAIN INGREDIENTS":

1. Water

2. Protein

3. Carbs

4. Fats

5. Fiber

6. Salt or Sodium

Dr. Dawn Psych MD's Tip:

Children react to foods differently. Some have allergic reactions to certain types of food (i.e., dairy, wheat, etc.) which can make ADHD symptoms worse.

Before you determine changes to your child's diet lifestyle, talk to your doctor about their recommendations.

Dr. Dawn Psych MD's Tip:

Being on a diet and maintaining a healthy nutritional lifestyle are very different. Here is a chart pointing out their major differences. Creating a healthy nutritional lifestyle is recommended.

	Diet	Healthy Nutritional Lifestyle
Time	Limited	Lifetime
Includes	Food only	Food, exercise, sleep hygiene
Cons	Risk for weight gain upon completion	Maintenance of a healthy weight (never completed)
	Usually eliminates less healthy foods	Includes less healthy foods at a minimal amount
Benefits	Short-lived and based on achievable weight goals	Long-term medical benefits

CHAPTER 5

The Recommended Balanced Diet – "What's on the Plate?"

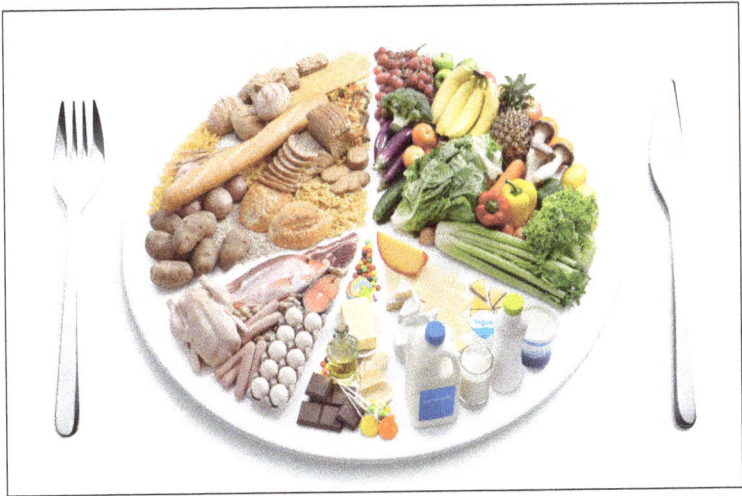

Eating a balanced diet means eating a variety of foods. Your child's plate should be "colorful"–– filled with foods from different food groups at recommended portions. A healthy meal consists of a balanced portion of vegetables, fruits, protein, carbohydrates, minerals, vitamins, and fat. There are also recommended portion sizes of each food group each day for children five to twelve years old.

1. **Veggies**   *Three Portions Daily*

   "Eat Your Vegetables! You Will Focus Longer and Remember More!"

   All veggies have polyphenols, which are known to be powerful antioxidants and assist with memory and cognition. Minerals, vitamins, and other plant nutrients aid your child's health by fighting off infection. Vitamin C creates a strong immune system and magnesium helps build healthy bones. Improve your child's chance of staying healthy by serving them carrots, tomatoes, zucchini, and corn. They'll thank you for it later!

2. **Fruit**   *Two Portions Daily*

   "An Apple at Night Will Keep ADHD Symptoms Packed Tight!"

   Doctors have recommended that children with ADHD increase their intake of complex carbohydrates (i.e., apples). Eating this fruit right before bed has been known to help children sleep better. Apples also help reduce bad breath; they are nature's breath freshener.

3. **Protein-rich foods** *Two Portions Daily*

"Protein is the BEST Fuel Source for the Brain!"

Meats, beans, cheese, eggs, and nuts contain good sources of protein. Give your young one these kinds of foods in the morning and as after-school snacks. They help improve concentration and possibly help ADHD medications work longer. They also help build muscles and help repair organs and glands.

4. **Grains and Potatoes** *Four-Six Portions Daily*

"The Essentials"

Provides energy, minerals, vitamins, carbohydrates, and iron.

Foods recommended that are rich in these fuel sources include breakfast cereals, breads, potatoes, rice, noodles, and pasta. These foods also provide your child with a good source of fiber to help with digestion and prevent constipation.

5. **Calcium-rich foods** *Two Portions Daily*

"Very Popular Among Kids!"

What kid doesn't want to grow up to be big and strong? Calcium plays a major role in building healthy bones and teeth. Foods containing a good amount of calcium include milk, cheese, and yogurt. But for the kids who don't like dairy foods or may have food allergies, which is common with many kids who have ADHD, calcium is also found in dark green leafy vegetables and beans.

6. **Healthy Fats and Oils**   *One Portion Daily*

"Healthy Fats Do Exist!"

Yes! You can find these in salmon, tuna, and other cold-water white fish. Walnuts, olive and canola oil are other foods that contain healthy fats. You could also give your child an omega-3 fatty acid supplement or the FDA approved omega compound, Vayarin, which is a medical food that is used in the management of ADHD. It is advised that you contact your child's doctor to find out if Vayarin is a good option. Vayarin is prescribed and cannot be purchased over the counter.

Question: Can eating salmon help improve learning behaviors?

Answer: Yes, because it contains a nutritional source of omega-3 fatty acids.

Question: Are vegetarians at a high risk of developing ADHD?

Answer: No. The lack of veggies in the diet does not cause ADHD. Rather, vegetables supply nutrients for the body's development and are most effective to help control ADHD symptoms when included in a well-balanced diet. Spinach is one of the most effective vegetables when considering ADHD symptom control.

Question: What is the difference between complex and simple carbohydrates?

Answer: Not all carbs are created equal.

Complex Carbs- These are the good guys. Load your kiddos up on vegetables and some fruits, including oranges, tangerines, pears, grapefruit, apples, and kiwi. These foods should be given in the evening, as they may help put your child to sleep. Although they contain natural sugars, too much of any food may not be healthy.

Simple Carbs- Closely monitor how much you allow your children to eat these guys: candy, sugar, honey, bleached foods (i.e., white flour, white rice), and potatoes without the skins. They often cause blood sugar spikes and crashes, leading to moodiness and crankiness. These "bad boys" are hard to digest when in abundance and may store as fat.

Dr. Dawn Psych MD's Tip:

Don't eliminate the carbohydrates! They are the body's MAIN fuel source and necessary for your health!

....

Foods to Avoid –
"Junk Food Swaps"

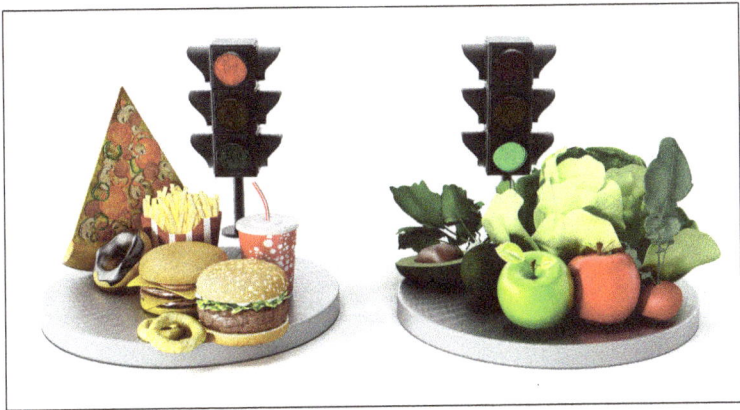

I remember my father picking me up from school and the next stop before home would be a food store where he would purchase a honey bun for me. He jokingly told me not to tell my mom, since he allowed me to eat it before dinner. Yet, the first thing I told my mom when I arrived home was that dad gave me a honey bun. Although my dad and I laugh about this memory today, we both understand Mom's conversations about why it is important to eat dinner before sweets. Her reason was to make sure that I had all of the required nutrients my growing body needed so that I could focus on my homework and chores.

For the child that has challenges with letting go of junk foods and a harder time with trying the healthy ones, be patient with them. Food marketing has made it difficult for a child with ADHD to avoid these foods at the end of the day when their medication has worn off. Considering the easy access kids have to junk food and how their impressionable minds are bombarded with snack TV ads, who could blame them? It is up to parents to regulate what their children eat, teach them healthy eating behaviors by prioritizing their nutritional intake, and allow them to practice what they have learned.

When considering food for your child's meals, it is important to recognize whether a product is high in certain ingredients or not by looking at its ingredients list. The list always starts with the biggest ingredient first then continues in descending order based on its amount. For example, if sugar is listed first, this tells you that the product contains high levels of sugar.

The following ingredients make products attractive to children's taste buds. Many are disguised in the foods that you may already have in your food cabinet.

1. Sugar

   It can be difficult to identify sugar, as it is called so many names on the ingredient list. Look for the names ending in "-ose:" glucose, fructose, sucrose, dextrose, and fruit syrup. They are all forms of sugar and can cause quick spikes and crashes in your ADHD child's behavior. Sugar is also not good for your child's teeth.

2. Hydrogenated Fats

   This artificially saturated fat is a processed fat and contains trans fats which are hard for your child's metabolism to break down, causing serious health risks. Instead of trans fat being written on labels, they are disguised as hydrogenated fats. They increase blood levels of the LDL ("Lousy") cholesterol and the risk of heart disease, stroke, diabetes, and certain cancers. Over the past 10 years, food companies have replaced hydrogenated fats with butter or healthy oils.

   It is advised to cut down on the following foods that contain high amounts of hydrogenated fats:

   a. Fast foods. Most are fried in variant amounts of hydrogenated oil.

   b. Chips and snacks.

   c. Chocolate bars. The vegetable fat listed on the label equals hydrogenated fat.

    d.   Cakes. Hydrogenated fat and shortening are used in cakes more than any other food.

    e.   Spreads made with hydrogenated oils. A good alternative is an olive oil spread.

3. Artificial Food Additives

Watch out for the additives! I tell parents in my practice that if you see an ingredient high on the list that is hard to pronounce, it is likely an **ADD**ITIVE!

Common additives:

    a.   Tartrazine (E102)

    b.   Sunset Yellow (E110)

    c.   Carmoisine (E122)

    d.   Ponceau (E124)

Question: Is it better to give children with ADHD sugar-free products that contain artificial sweeteners instead of sugar?

Answer: No. Ironically, some studies show that artificial sweeteners can increase your child's urges for real sugar. Artificial sweeteners have also been known to cause cancer in laboratory mice.

THE HIDDEN SUGARS

Look out for them! They are disguised on Nutritional Information lists as: glucose, dextrose, fruit syrup, and glucose syrup. ALL sugars damage teeth, increase blood sugar levels, and cause inflammation, a spike in the insulin peak, and weight gain.

JUNK FOOD SWAPS

Replace:	With:
Crisps or Salty Packet Snacks	Plain popcorn, low-fat baked potato chips, mini rice cakes
Biscuits or White Flour Products	Rice cakes with peanut butter, fig rolls
Shop-bought Cakes	Whole wheat hot cross bun or fruit bun
Sweets	Packet of dried fruit or nuts, pre-made fruit salad
Chocolate Bars	Cereal, nut, or fruit bar
Soda Pops	Water, fruit juice (ideally diluted 50/50), low-fat milk, smoothie

Dr. Dawn Psych MD's Tip:

So, here's an obvious fact: junk food is really bad for kids with ADHD. Many parents avoid buying them because junk foods, like sweets, can cause an over-active child to become more over-active. The truth of the matter is this likely occurs when kids choose to eat sweets over foods that provide important minerals, vitamins, and fiber, resulting in them missing out on the healthy nutrients their body needs. I can't imagine life for a child without sweets. Once they have met their daily nutritional needs for fruits, grains, healthy fats, vegetables, calcium-rich and protein-rich foods, then it is okay for them to have a sweet treat.

CHAPTER 7

Getting Kids with ADHD to Eat Fruits and Veggies – "I Don't Want to Eat That!"

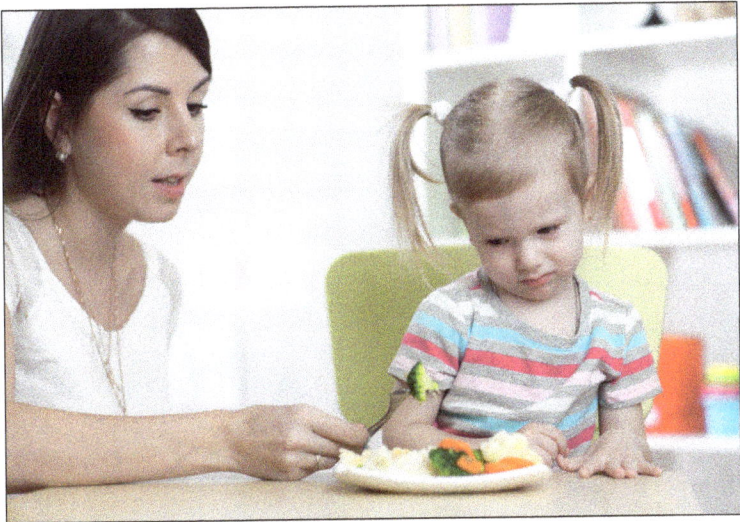

I laugh when I think back to my mom making me eat my vegetables when I was younger. I would often pout when I saw broccoli or spinach on my plate, especially if it touched Mom's famous fried chicken or mac and cheese. I would hide a few veggies in my napkin and throw them away. This stopped when my mom finally caught me and for a period of time served my veggies first before I could eat my meats. I remember Mom saying, "Dawn, eat your veggies. They are healthy for you. They help with your memory and aid in your digestion." I disliked veggies because I thought they looked and tasted nasty. She helped me to eventually enjoy them by putting them with other foods I liked (i.e., tomatoes on hamburgers) or adding flavor to them by using other ingredients (i.e., broccoli with cheese). I now understand why veggies are crucial for my nutrition and mentation. And, I now truly appreciate my mom's early lessons.

Most kids want a say in what they eat; they want the option to choose. As Mom, you control what is on the list and they can choose from that list.

Tip 1: Have your child pick three veggies and two fruits.

Create a list of the fruits and vegetables that your child enjoys. Encourage your child to pick one fruit and vegetable they haven't tried or don't commonly eat to avoid the boredom of the same foods.

Tip 2: Create a "5-a-day plan" routine.

Have your child choose three vegetables and two fruits from a list every day. These food items can be eaten between two to three meals, but may be easier when incorporated into three meals and two snacks.

Tip 3: Teach your child to eat five different colors of fruits and vegetables. For example:

Green- Spinach, Greens, Beans

Red- Tomatoes, Apples, Red Cabbage

Yellow- Squash, Corn, Bananas

Orange- Oranges, Carrots, Sweet Potatoes

Brown- Mushrooms, Raisins

Tip 4: Set the example.

Your child is very impressionable during their younger years, which allow routines to be easily followed but may be more of a challenge for caregivers to maintain. If you have established these routines in your personal life, it is likely easy to do the same for your child's lifestyle. Don't forget to be consistent, and remember it usually takes three weeks to three months to establish and maintain a routine.

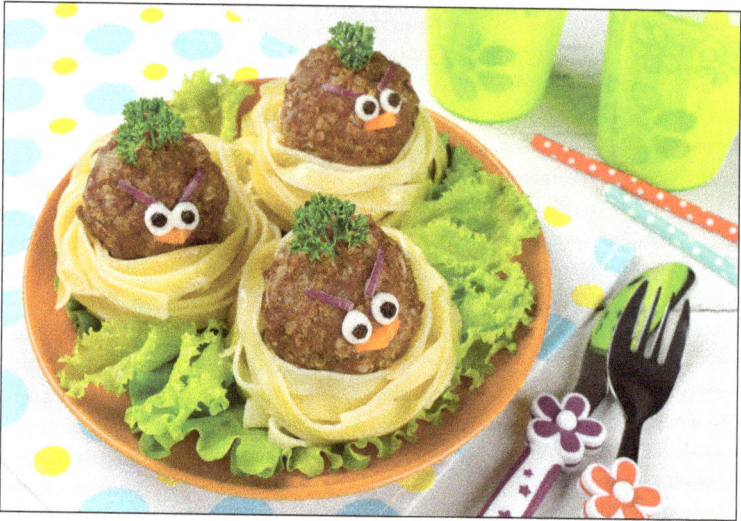

Tip 5: Make it FUN!

Here are some fun ideas to make vegetables and fruits enjoyable for your child to eat:

a.   Grow your own vegetables and fruits.

b.   Allow your kids to help prepare family meals by including their daily required foods from which they can choose. Suggest that they help you pick them out at the grocery store.

c.   Gradually add vegetables and fruits to what they already enjoy (i.e., toppings on pizza, ingredients for a protein shake).

d. Let them choose from your pre-selection of vegetables and fruits (start small).

e. Hide them within food (i.e., blended shakes).

f. Start *fruits early in the day (i.e., as a breakfast item).

g. Have *fruits for dinner (sweet tastes decrease hunger and curbs the appetite).

*Studies have shown that some fruits may help with digestion.

Jazz up the veggie appeal by creating funny items, objects, and faces on the plate (Pinterest has some really neat ideas on how to do this)!

Dr. Dawn Psych MD's Tip:

Place a bowl filled with fruit in areas where your kids can reach them. They will likely grab a fruit for a snack or to eat while dinner is being prepared.

CHAPTER 8

The Grocery List – "Shopping for Groceries with Your ADHD Child"

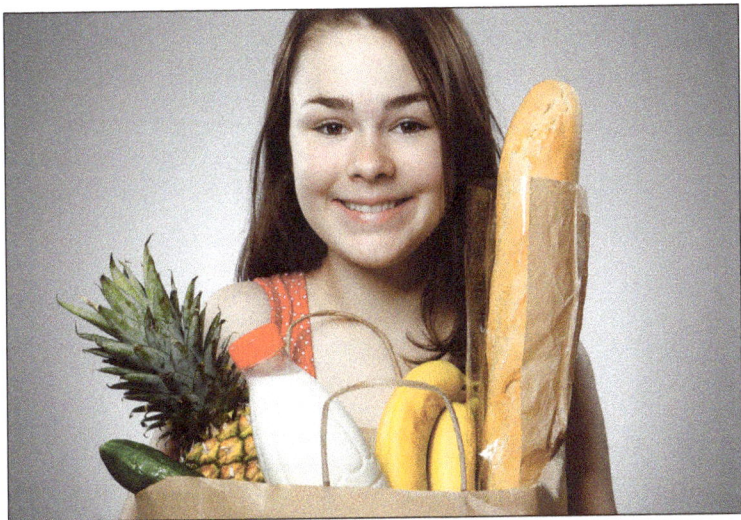

Shopping for groceries with your ADHD child can be one of the biggest challenges a mom faces. Using behavior management strategies and involving your child in the shopping routine can help guide them through the experience but also nurture them to choose healthy food options. Before you take a trip to the store, review The Five P's to make the most of grocery shopping!

Avoid displays at the ends of aisles and while in the check-out line. They are intentionally located to increase impulsive buying (which is not good for impulsive symptoms of ADHD).

1. **The PREPARER**- Make a shopping list. Place it on the fridge for everyone to view. If it's not on the list, don't buy it!

2. **The PLANNER**- YOU are in charge. YOU have the cash. Consider setting time limits in the store.

3. **The PARTNER**- Allow your children to help. Read the item and help them locate it. If another caregiver goes, split the list.

4. **The PROTECTOR**- Avoid shopping when hungry. Eat before you shop. Hungry people buy more food, especially junk food.

5. **The PERIMETER**- Shop LESS in the middle of the store, which mostly includes aisles of sweets, preservatives, chips, and sugary drinks. Shop the perimeter for fresh vegetables, fruits, and perishable foods.

Avoid times when the grocery store is crowded. This will decrease distractibility and allow good use of time management practices, with intentions of sticking to the items on your list.

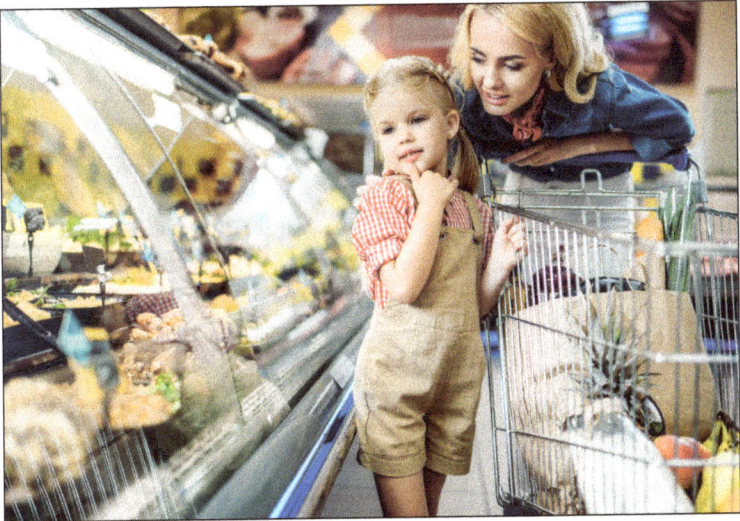

Use shopping apps to help organize your grocery list and coupons.

Dr. Dawn Psych MD's Tip:

An alternative to buying organic foods would be to thoroughly wash your fruits and vegetables, which removes some of the pesticide residue. Peeling does the same.

Consider the grocery store shopping service that gathers groceries and provides curbside pick-up for a fee.

CHAPTER 9

The Most Important Meal of the Day- "Break-Your-FAST!"

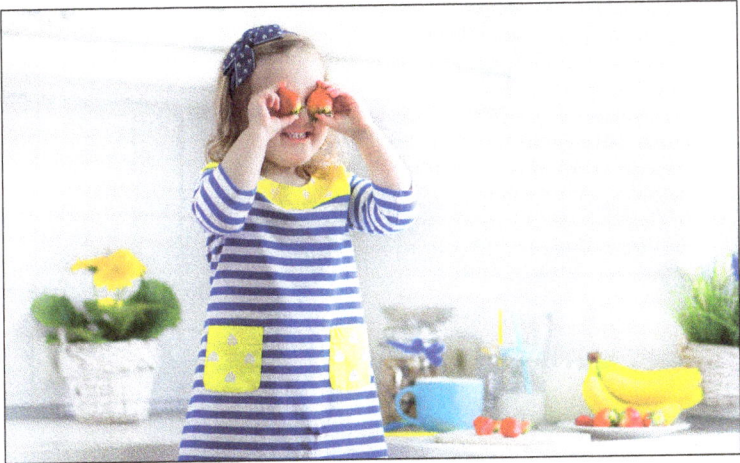

I recall my mother fixing oatmeal for breakfast before I went to school. Growing up in Michigan, most of the year was cold months and oatmeal was the perfect choice, especially for those breezy winter days. My mom routinely expressed that breakfast was the most important meal of the day. And although the phrase may be considered a cliché, she was correct! Breakfast provides us with the energy to get our day started and gives clarity to our thoughts. I can still hear my mom say, "Dawn, you need to break-your-fast! You haven't eaten since yesterday and I know your brain and stomach are hungry!" My mom was a very smart woman and she knew exactly what my body needed.

1. WHY is breakfast important?

   a. "Feeds your personality."

   b. Creates better moods.

   c. Provides longer focus and sustained attention.

   d. Increases energy levels and motivation.

   e. Enhances learning abilities.

   f. Helps to reduce the side effect profile of a stimulant medication.

2. Eat simple, high-protein meals for breakfast.

   a. Includes vegetable and fruit servings.

   b. Helps medication be more effective.

   c. Food examples: eggs, whole grain cereals, oatmeal, yogurt, diced fruits.

   d. Helps with digestion and makes metabolism more efficient.

3. Eat whole and minimally processed foods.

   a. Easier to break down.

   b. Less salt included in minimally processed foods.

   c. Minimal to no additives (additives can cause food sensitivities).

   d. Contains a greater source of nutrients that are often lost in processed foods.

4. Avoid frozen breakfast foods and high sugary foods (i.e., donuts, pastries, and high sugary cereals).

Dr. Dawn Psych MD's Tip:

Preservatives are found in processed foods and can be unhealthy for your child's wellbeing. They contain fillers that are not real food, which decreases the likelihood of your child eating their daily nutritional requirements.

CHAPTER 10

The Importance of School Lunches – "The ADHD Lunchbox"

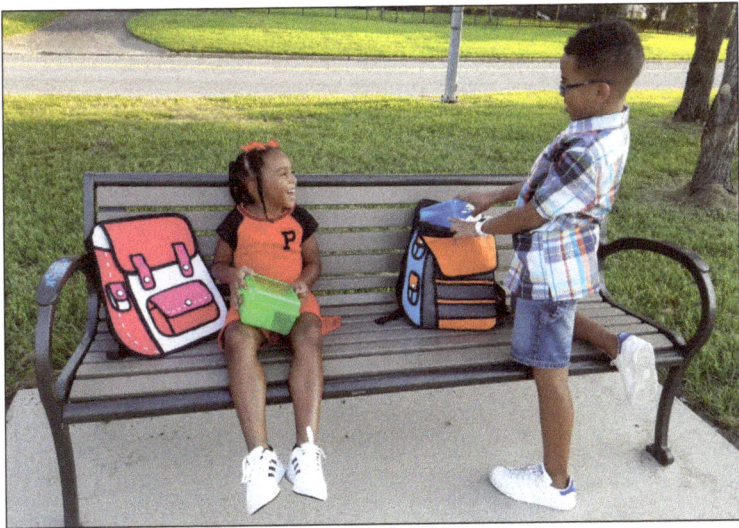

Lunchtime can be a difficult experience for kids with ADHD. Kids have a challenging time with eating their lunch, usually because their medication causes a decrease in their appetite. To make matters worse, many kids are either uncomfortable about eating in a noisy and well-populated lunch room or stimulated by the environment; therefore, making their way around the cafeteria to catch up with friends.

Another major reason why kids, in general, do not eat during lunch is because of the food their school serves. Prior to the success of the Obama Administration's creation of the Healthy, Hunger-Free Kids Act, school lunches were discovered to contain high amounts of sodium and trans fats, and less than the recommended age-appropriate nutritional servings of vegetables, fruits, and whole grains.

It is also important to recognize the association between a well-balanced meal and academic success. It can be challenging for a child who is hungry or does not eat a well-nourished meal to effectively learn in the classroom.

So, how do we tackle these concerns for children who live with ADHD? What can be done to increase the likelihood that a child with ADHD eats their lunch?

I always encourage my patients to eat something, even if they are not hungry, during their lunchtime. Eating something will help stimulate their appetite, combating the potential appetite suppressant that stimulant medications could cause. I also educate children and their caregivers that the appetite suppressant side effect usually takes time to resolve. Finally, I discuss with children and their parents the ideal foods they enjoy, and from that list, I help them choose healthy foods to include in their ADHD Lunch Box. I ask parents, "Would you rather your child consume a homemade lunch or a preservative-laden school lunch? Are you aware of the ingredients in school lunches?" Last, I discuss the importance of planning if their child decides to take a lunch to school.

I created an ADHD Lunch Box that provides ADHD elementary students with a food container that features dividers and compartments that can conveniently store the basic nutritional food requirements that I recommend for ADHD children of different age groups. It can be purchased on www.drdawnpsychmd.com.

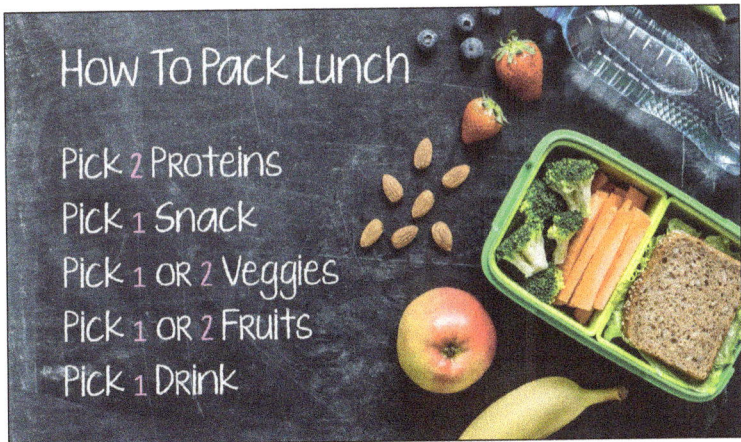

How To Pack Lunch

Pick 2 Proteins
Pick 1 Snack
Pick 1 OR 2 Veggies
Pick 1 OR 2 Fruits
Pick 1 Drink

Packing a Healthy Lunch Box:

1. 1/3 of daily energy requires 1/3 of protein, carbs, fiber, vitamin, and mineral needs.

    a. 200-300 ml drink: water or juice

    b. 1 portion of fresh or dried fruit

    c. 1 portion of salad, veggies, or carrot sticks

    d. 1 carb: bread, roll, or pasta

    e. 1 dairy or calcium-enriched item

    f. 1 protein-enriched meat or fish, peanut butter, hummus egg

Dr. Dawn Psych MD's Tip:

Use leftover dinner meals for lunch the following day.

Avoid all-in-one lunch meals, which are targeted at young kids. Most contain high levels of fillers, saturated fats, and preservatives, and don't provide much vitamins or fiber.

Example of a home prepared lunch meal plan for one week of school

Monday	Tuesday	Wednesday
Dry fruit	Apple	Pear
Carrot sticks	Cucumber sticks	Salad
PB&J sandwich	Turkey Sandwich	Mini Pita bread
Low-fat yogurt	Fruit muffins	Hardboiled egg
Water	Chocolate milk	Low-fat milk

Thursday	Friday
Banana	Fresh Fruit
Hummus	Salad
Sliced carrots	Mini Bagel
Individual cheese	Chopped chicken
Diluted Fruit Juice	Whole milk

* Snacks can include: beef jerky, whole grain protein bars, apple slices, unsalted nuts, peanut butter and celery sticks.

Lunch should aim to supply the following requirements. If it doesn't, make sure the requirements are included in your child's snacks or at dinner.

1. 1/3 of the daily energy requirements

2. 1/3 of carbohydrate, protein, fiber, vitamin, and mineral requirements

Dr. Dawn Psych MD's Tip:

Moms, I am sure you are amazed at what your child can do, especially at an early age. Five and six-year-olds may be opening the fridge and getting snacks from the shelves, so packing a lunch would naturally be the next step in the adventure!

Here is a helpful way to begin teaching your young one independence while you maintain control over the choices they make.

This pictorial provides your child with food options from each food group, allowing them to make healthy lunch choices.

A convenient place to hang this image would be on the family fridge or an area for your child to easily view. You and your child can also have fun creating your own drawings after teaching them about healthy food lunch items.

HOW TO PACK LUNCH

pick 2 proteins

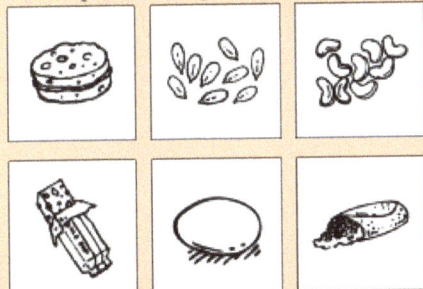

pick a drink

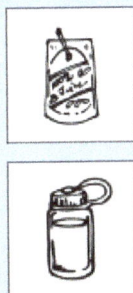

pick 1 snack

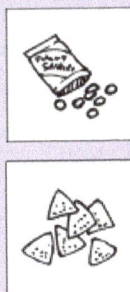

pick 1 or 2 veggies

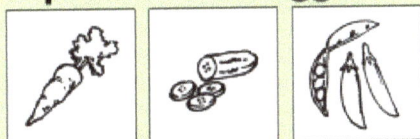

pick 1 or 2 fruits

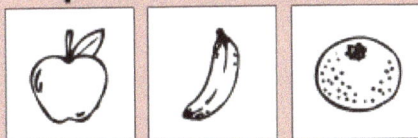

CHAPTER 11

Dinnertime!
Kids in the Kitchen –
"Fun with Food"

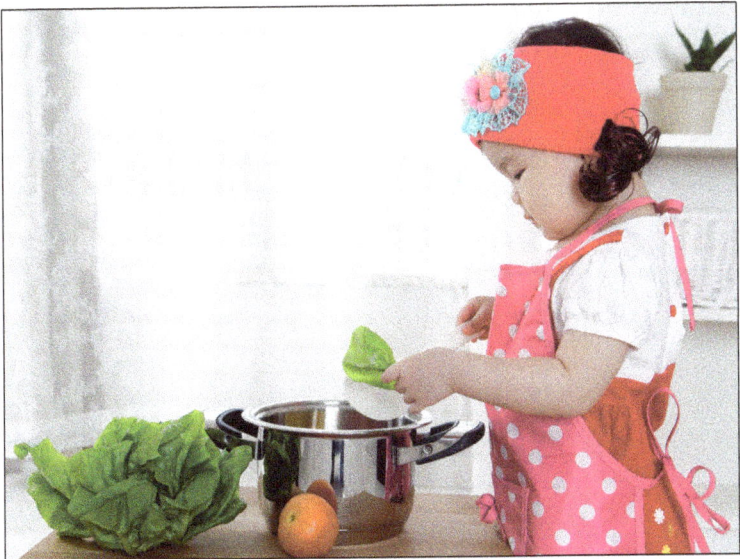

Cooking can be great fun for children with ADHD, even during the early evenings when their symptoms can be more challenging to manage. The undercelebrated traits of a child with ADHD—creativity, innovation, imagination, and intelligence can be valuable in the kitchen! When your child steps into your kitchen, another superpower emerges. Creating their own dishes gives them a sense of achievement and can be a way to motivate picky eaters to try new tastes and gain confidence with the food they helped to create. Preparing meals can also provide an educational experience; children often learn new skills fast when they have a desired interest. They'll learn about what's healthy versus unhealthy, weighing, measuring, mixing, spreading, cutting, organizing, and how to follow and improvise recipe instructions. They will also learn a little bit of chemistry—how ingredients work together and what food groups go well together.

Considering the fast-paced world we live in, prepping for dinner can also be a dedicated time for parents to spend valuable time with their kids. The conversation can also continue around the dinner table, where parents learn about their child's day at school, their friendships, and their personal accomplishments.

When preparing meals, I encourage you to consider the following recommendations to create a fun and safe kitchen experience for your child:

1. **Assign meal prep tasks that are developmentally relevant and age-appropriate for your child.**

   I remember when my mom first taught me how to cook. I was a curious and impressionable seven-year-old who dreamed of cooking like her. She could make tasty and flavorful dishes in no time! She first taught me how to scramble eggs. Our version may be different from yours because instead of beginning the mixture process in a separate bowl, we scrambled the egg contents in a hot skillet. I am not certain if my mom knew that I had ADHD, but my impulsive energy and enthusiastic personality (aka: ADHD symptoms) might have led her to skip the first step and start in the pan! LOL! Nevertheless, I'd like to think my mom created a way for me to cook without focusing on or pointing out my unmanaged symptoms. Till this day, I create my eggs the same way.

2. **Tasking your child to help with meal prep creates confidence, increases the odds of tasting what they cooked, and may even lead to a future talent!**

   As mentioned in a previous chapter, I despised broccoli. I also hated salad. I know these may be strong words, but I was born a meat eater. Meats were the first and last tastes in my mouth whenever I ate a meal. My favorite meat is still fried chicken! When I think of how moist and flavorful each bite of my mom's famous friend chicken tasted, I can't help but to love it! I used to ask her if I could sample a wing or two whenever she was cooking; she never said no. But, when the veggie dish touched the sides of my chicken, I remember thinking, "Why do I have to eat something that does not taste good, changes the flavor of whatever it touches, and looks nasty?" I am sure many of you Moms have probably heard these excuses after placing a serving on your child's plate. But, my mom was creative with getting me to start liking salad. Not only did she add fried chicken, but she assigned me to cut up the salad's ingredients, while educating me on the importance of each vegetable's role on my body! I recall some of the things she used to say when I was young:

"Dawn, it is important to eat your carrots because they help with your vision at night."

"It's important that you eat green vegetables because they help your gut digest your food (keeps you regular)."

"Eating vegetables helps your brain think better, provides energy for your body, and creates happy thoughts and moods."

The addition of fried chicken and cut vegetables on my salad had a meaningful impact, as it has become a common dish of mine when I prepare my own meals or when I order from a restaurant menu. Adding your child's favorite food item to a meal can increase the likelihood that they may enjoy it, especially if they helped prepare it!

3. **Use and appreciate your child's imagination and creativity in the meal prep process.**

This will allow your child to become more knowledgeable about herbs, spices, mixtures, and ingredients while utilizing the rebound ADHD symptoms to their benefit during dinner prep. Allowing their imagination reinforces their abilities and increases their confidence. Mixing, blending, measuring, substituting, baking, and any other cooking activities allows you to provide valuable teaching moments, which are reinforced by hands-on experimentation. It can also be a neat idea for a child to understand the difference between baking soda and baking powder and how this difference impacts the result. Many chefs and culinary experts will tell you that they also learned by following recipes and creating different dishes on their own.

If you find the time, it would be a neat experience for you and your child to create your own individual dishes that include the same ingredients. Create a friendly competition!

Try the recipes in Chapter 16. They are easy enough for older children to make on their own. The younger children may need help from an adult.

CHAPTER 12

Healthy Snacks and ADHD – "Stay Alert and Keep Calm"

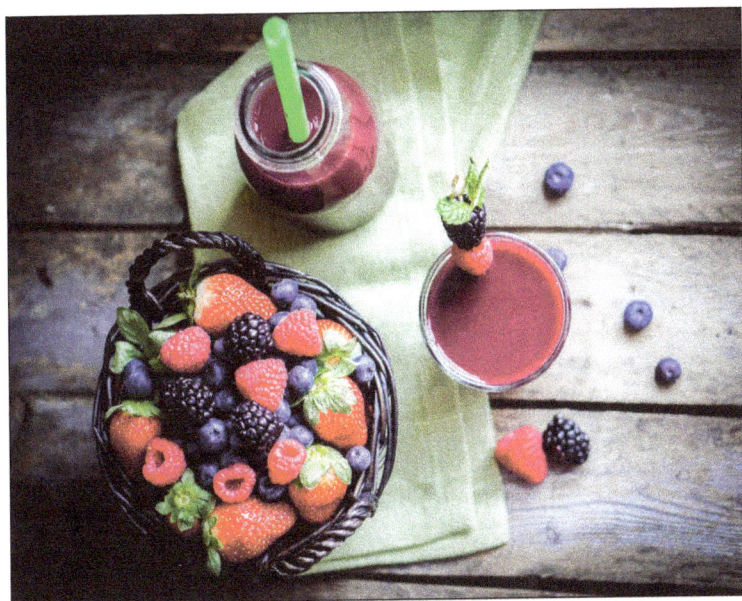

It is important for kids to maintain healthy diet lifestyles as they grow and develop. Snacks, like meals, are just as important to include in their regimen. Kids with ADHD have challenges with meal consistency for many reasons:

1. Stimulant medications can suppress their appetite, often leaving kids hungry at inconvenient times.

2. A child's hyperactivity may release more energy and require more calories in comparison to their peers (without ADHD).

3. If kids eat more sweets in their diet as a snack, children with ADHD appear moodier when blood sugar spikes and then crashes.

Food marketing has gone to great lengths to find the right tools to capture your child's attention. For example, timely commercials, marketing location in the store, and packaging are three important concepts that food companies spend billions of dollars on that would likely lead to a successful sale of their products. I believe snacks not only have the most impact on our kids, but they are the biggest threat to healthy eating, as many snacks are pre-packaged and filled with preservatives, fillers, and sugar but not enough of the nutrients, minerals, and vitamins that a child needs. Pre-packaged items such as chips, fruit cups, and fruit snacks may be easy to purchase and pick up before running out the door; however, the healthiest snacks are the snacks that are homemade.

DR. DAWN PSYCH MD'S RECIPE FOR "A VERY BERRY SMOOTHIE" (2 SERVINGS)

Prep time: 2 minutes

Blending time: 3 minutes

Ready in: 5 minutes

This recipe is rich in antioxidants and contains high amounts of vitamin C and phytochemicals, which have protective and disease preventive properties. Ingredients:

1. 8-ounce bag of mixed fresh or frozen berries of your choice (i.e., strawberries, raspberries, blueberries, blackberries). Set aside 2 tablespoons of berries

2. 4-ounce carton of strawberry probiotic yogurt

3. 8 fluid ounces of milk

Instructions:

1. Place all ingredients into a smoothie maker, blender, or food processor and blend until smooth.

2. Place 2 tablespoons of the berries you set aside on top of your smoothie and ENJOY!

Here's a list of healthy snacks you can encourage your child to eat after school, but before dinner. Keep in mind that protein is the best fuel source for the brain.

1. Veggie sticks with dip or peanut butter

2. Dried fruits or nuts

3. Cereal bars

4. Hummus

5. Fruit shakes or smoothies (Dr. Dawn Psych MD's FAVORITE recipe)

6. PB&J

7. Pretzels or whole wheat crackers

8. Mini pizzas

CHAPTER 13

Boost Your Brain Power – "Exercise Your Mind"

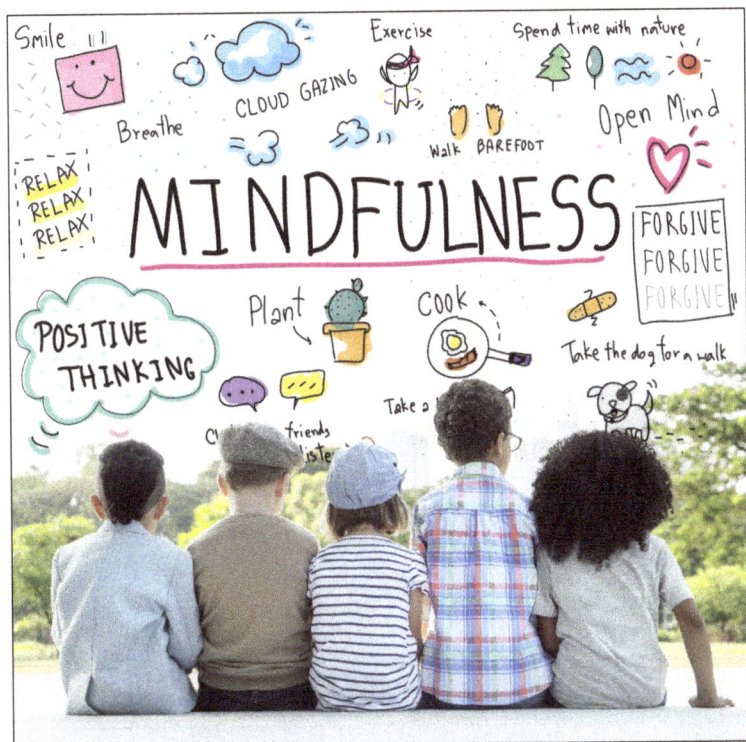

When the word exercise is mentioned, it is uncommon for a person to think about mental exercises, particularly for kids. Physical activity is a part of a child's routine. Running, jumping, skipping, and hopping are forms of exercise that allow the body to develop muscle strengthening, coordination, and gets the heart pumping and the circulation going. However, brain exercises have been shown to be used as an adjunct behavior technique to assist with providing better impulse control, improving focus and memory, and calming a hyperactive mind. These, in turn, help children strategize, organize, memorize, and process information.

Has your child left the math book at school that is needed to complete homework? Does your child re-read paragraphs several times to recall what was read? Has your child repeatedly left their lunchbox on the kitchen table? Some may think these are typical signs of inattention, but they are likely deficits of working memory. Short-term memory is often used interchangeably with working memory, which are brief thoughts that are held in your mind and used to complete tasks. Studies show that a child's working memory capacity is limited to remembering one or two words. This memory type develops until around age 15, but not all children grow at the same pace. Improving your child's working memory enhances their ability to problem solve and increases their processing speed and memory adaptability. Our working memory is essential for both school and everyday life because it involves our ability to organize, read, write, complete math problems, and follow multi-step directions. It can increase your child's alertness to social cues.

Some examples of games that can help improve your child's working memory and brain power are the classics: Simon, Memory flashcards, and Sudoku. These games incorporate memory skills, math, and logic. They can increase a child's working memory capacity during gameplay, but this decreases when the game ends. There are significant improvements in working memory when these games become routine in your child's schedule.

When we are less stressed, the brain can process information better, we experience calmer emotions, and we make healthy decisions. Mindfulness meditation also achieves this. Mindfulness is being aware of our present thoughts and feelings while having the ability to refocus when we become distracted. With an ADHD child, the state of mindfulness is accomplished by teaching your child to focus on his breathing pattern and notice that there is a silence that exists between inhaling and exhaling. Although this concept has other elements involved, the goal is for a child to be aware of their thoughts and feelings and choose to make the right decisions. Mindfulness has a positive impact on our moods and helps decrease anxiety, anger, and depression while improving attention, sleep hygiene, and mood behaviors. It is an essential brain power tool that is used to help manage ADHD symptoms.

Dr. Dawn Psych MD's Tip:

Limit screen times for kids with ADHD. It can be tough for any child to turn off their electronic devices, but it can be extremely challenging for kids with ADHD to detach from their devices. This is partly due to TV rays (that cannot be seen by the human eye) which act similar to stimulants by increasing your child's focus.

You decide on customary times when your child uses electronics. I have recommended to my patients with ADHD (children and adults) that they turn off electronics at least one hour before their bedtime. Consider asking your pediatrician or child psychiatrist for their behavior management recommendations for screen time and proper sleep hygiene relative to your child's age group.

Ask about recommended screen times for:

1. TV

2. Computer

3. Tablet

4. Gaming

5. Phone

Dr. Dawn Psych MD's Tip:

Keep in mind: Quality > Quantity.

The quality of what your child views is more important than the quantity of how much they watch. Talk to your child about the programs, websites, games, or apps you have determined are appropriate for their viewing.

CHAPTER 14

The Colorful Healthy Plate – "Healthy Meal Ideas for an Active Mind"

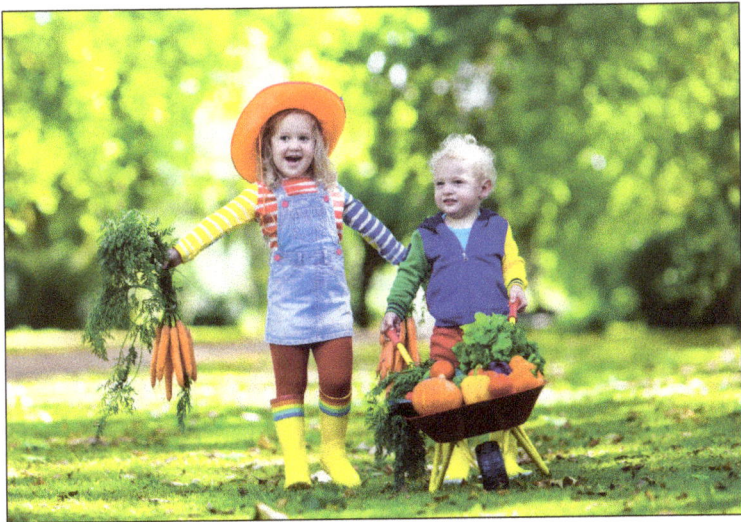

Have you heard the saying, "Variety is the spice of life?" Well, no pun intended. When considering meals for kids with

ADHD, having variety can help create new and exciting experiences for a child's appetite, especially when their appetite fluctuates depending on the timing of their medications or based on their activity levels when compared with their peers without ADHD. Having a variety of options also prevents boredom, which is important for an active mind.

Variety is the key to creating and maintaining healthy meals for balanced eating. These menus include the dietary recommendations from MyPyramid and provide a good balance of protein, carbohydrates, vitamins, minerals, and fat.

Here are two full-day menus for five- to ten-year-olds and eleven- to 15-year-olds, to include a vegetarian full day menu for both groups. Determine the portion sizes according to your child's age group, activity, and appetite.

And don't forget the fluids! Encourage your kids to drink at least six to eight glasses of fluid (water, milk, diluted fruit juice) daily, and more during exercise or when playing outside in hot climates.

MEAL DAY PLAN
(FIVE- TO TEN-YEAR-OLDS)

Breakfast	Whole wheat cereal with milk Banana
Lunch	Tuna with low-fat mayo on wheat bread Small ring-pull cup of fruit in juice (no sugar added) Yogurt cup Water
Snack	Veggie sticks with peanut butter
Dinner	Grilled chicken burgers **Oven wedged potatoes Baked Beans or broccoli Stewed or sliced apples (a breath freshener!)

MEAL DAY PLAN
(ELEVEN- TO FIFTEEN-YEAR-OLDS)

Breakfast	**Strawberry and Banana Smoothie Banana
Lunch	Bagel with low-fat cheese and tuna Small bag of nuts and raisins Fresh fruits Water
Snack	Blueberry or apple muffins

Dinner   Grilled Salmon, topped with parsley and basil
Broccoli and Carrots
Rice Pilaf

VEGETARIAN MEAL DAY PLAN (FIVE- TO TEN-YEAR-OLDS)

Breakfast   Wholegrain cereal with milk
Orange Juice

Lunch   Bean Burger
Wheat roll
Fruit
Yogurt cup
Water

Snack   **Gingerbread cookies

Dinner   Macaroni and Cheese with peas
Green beans and carrots
Rice pudding with fresh fruit

VEGETARIAN MEAL DAY PLAN (ELEVEN- TO FIFTEEN-YEAR-OLDS)

Breakfast   English muffin or bagel
Fresh fruit

Lunch   **Bean and Tuna salad
Yogurt

	Seedless grapes
	Water
Snack	Protein bars with chocolate chips
Dinner	Potato filled with stir-fried vegetables or
	Ratatouille
	Apple crumble
	Custard or yogurt

**Recipe found in Chapter 16

CHAPTER 15

Benefits of Activity for a Busy Mind – "Let's Stay Active!"

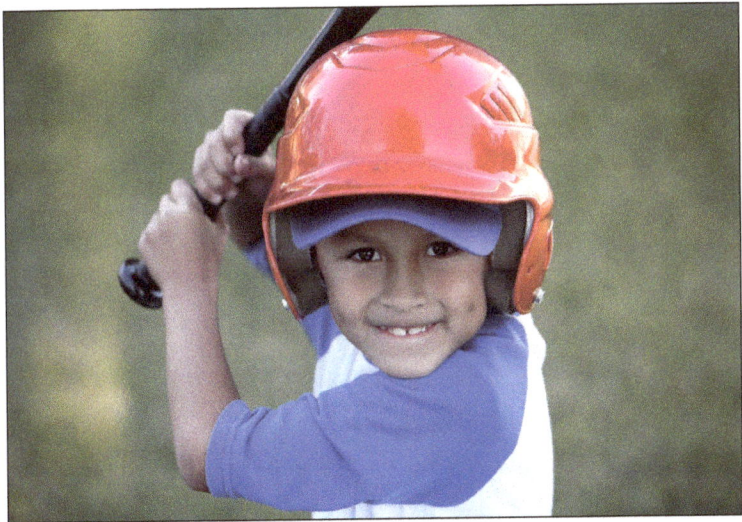

Exercise benefits the heart. It builds stronger muscles. It increases flexibility. It boosts the mood and decreases worry. It keeps the weight down and can improve concentration and reasoning.

So, WHY is it challenging at times for children with ADHD to exercise?! Well, recreational activities and organized sports often take place in the early evenings when kids with ADHD are less focused and may require adult supervision. During this time of day, medications are no longer at therapeutic levels in their system and begin to wear off, resulting in ADHD symptoms returning.

It is important to discuss with your psychiatrist your observations of your child's attention span, activity or energy levels, and degree of impulse control during the early evenings. There are times when medication adjustments and additions must be made to obtain greater symptom control. Exercise has also been found to enhance medications' effectiveness for ADHD symptom control and plays a vital role in releasing endorphins—"the happy hormones" that help create happy moods. The combination of exercise and medication prevents your child from becoming distracted, helps them maintain a safe outlook, and improves their engagement level with friends. They are also more apt to follow their coach's instructions, and their chance of performing close to their optimal skill level is increased.

Not all activities are age appropriate. Caution should be considered when deciding at what age your child is physically and emotionally ready for various levels of recreational activities and organized sports.

A. Activities for children less than twelve years of age should focus on ENJOYMENT.

B. Activities for children more than twelve years of age should provide a variety of sports options (i.e., dance, gymnastics) to develop a good range of movement skills and enhance mobility.

C. Specialized sports should not be considered until age 11.

The Recommended Amount of Exercise for Kids (grouped by age range):

1. Ages Two to Five

   Play daily. Focus on developing basic skills such as running, jumping, and coordination.

   a. Playing tag

   b. Skipping

   c. Swimming

   d. Playing catch

   e. Riding a bike

2. Ages Six to Ten

   Require at least 60 minutes of moderate and intense activity daily.

a. Playground games

b. Hide and seek

c. Dancing

d. *Gymnastics

e. *Martial Arts

*Recommended at least twice weekly; enhances strength, flexibility, and bone health.

3. Ages Eleven to Fifteen

At least 30-60 minutes of moderate activity daily.

a. Team sports (**football, basketball, **rugby, and **hockey)

b. Tennis

c. Cycling

d. Running or Jogging

e. In-line skating

**Appropriate safety gear to protect your child from head to toe is essential. Make sure you are aware of what your child needs before they start!

It's important to establish a routine. Build activity into your family's daily routine so all members can benefit from FUN, heart-healthy activity while enjoying time together.

1. Find activities children can do with their parents (biking, walking, playing catch, throwing a frisbee).

2. Add purpose to the activities (walking the dog, practicing for school sports team).

3. Lead by example (value activities by consistently participating with your kids).

4. Encourage a wide range of activities or sports (to prevent boredom, which ADHD kids often report. Allows them to learn and develop movement skills).

5. Keep it FUN (be enthusiastic, give praise).

6. Make the activity sociable with their friends.

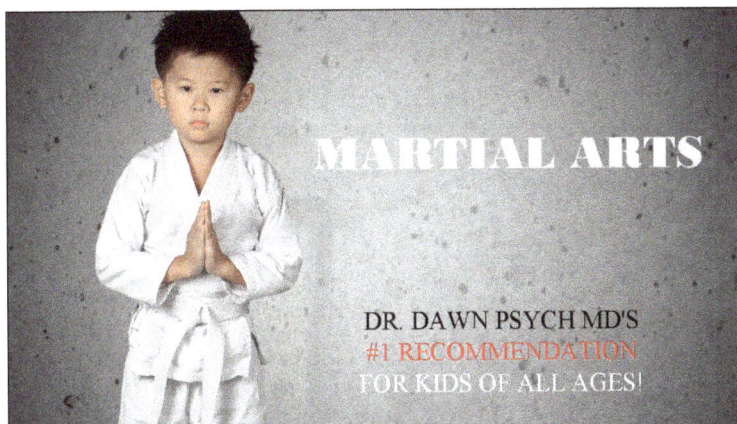

MARTIAL ARTS

DR. DAWN PSYCH MD'S
#1 RECOMMENDATION
FOR KIDS OF ALL AGES!

Examples of after-school activities:

1. Martial Arts (Dr. Dawn Psych MD's FAVORITE to recommend!)

   Young kids can participate (not advocated for competition until age 12).

   a. Teaches discipline.

   b. Creates and maintains a healthy heart.

   c. Results in increased blood flow to the brain.

   d. Recognized as a regimented sport.

   e. Includes achievement belts.

   f. Teaches self-defense (boosts confidence).

   g. Provides individual attention and practice.

   h. Provides incremental awards or achievements.

   i. Creates friendships or peer support.

   j. Groups by rank (safe and appropriate).

   k. Involves competition while respecting the opponent.

   l. Teaches regimen or structure.

   m. Helps with muscle strengthening and coordination.

    n.   Shares values that hopefully mesh with your family's values.

2.   Scouting troops

3.   Team sports

4.   Art and Music classes

OTHER EXAMPLES OF AFTER-SCHOOL ACTIVITIES

❯ Walk at least 20 minutes a day

❯ Play with family members or friends

❯ Gardening or yard work with caregivers

❯ Hiking or backpacking

❯ Outdoor sports

❯ Fishing

❯ Play frisbee with animals or walk pets

Dr. Dawn Psych MD's Safety Tips:

1.   Wear a helmet when riding bikes.

2.   Use all protective gear (helmets, pads, etc.) when playing tag football, etc.

3. Play in safe areas or parks.

4. Make sure children have adequate supervision.

5. Adhere to doctor's visits and recommendations.

Activities don't just take place outside. Make your child's household chores FUN by creating a scheduled plan with them for when and how to complete their daily and weekly tasks. Put this plan on the refrigerator for the entire family to view. Consider creating a chore check off list so that the child can learn time management, prioritize tasks, and feel accomplished and needed in the maintenance of the household.

Daily and weekly routines:

Weekly chores can be assigned if you have more than one child (i.e., Daily: make bed or clean room. Weekly: set dishes on table, take out trash, gardening).

CHAPTER 16

Recipes Created by Kids from Dr. Dawn Psych MD's Practice – "Kids' Kitchen"

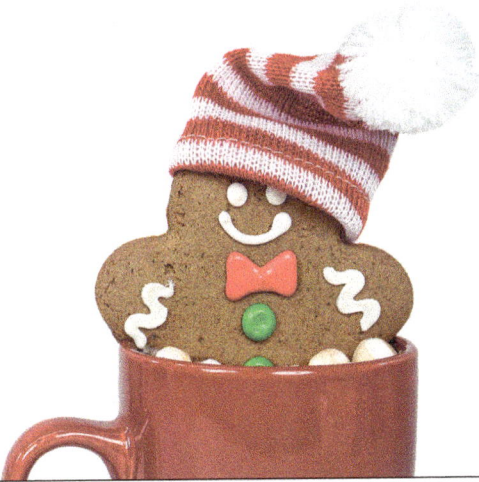

OVEN POTATO WEDGES (4 SERVINGS)

Created by Dylan

Prep time: 10 minutes
Cook time: 25 minutes
Ready in: 35 minutes

This recipe includes a good source of complex carbohydrates, fiber, and vitamin C.

Ingredients:

1. 4 large potatoes (or 2 russet potatoes), scrubbed and cut into eighths

2. 1 tablespoon of olive oil

3. 1 teaspoon of onion powder

4. 1 teaspoon of garlic powder

5. ¼ cup of parmesan cheese

6. ¼ teaspoon of ground black pepper

7. ¼ teaspoon of salt

8. Seasonings (optional): garlic powder, chili powder, and parmesan cheese

Instructions:

1. Preheat oven to 425 degrees F (220 degrees C).

2. Place ALL ingredients into a plastic bag.

3. Seal, then shake the bag so that the potatoes are fully coated with the seasoning.

4. Place the potatoes over a baking sheet.

5. Bake in the oven for 25 minutes or until the potatoes are soft and can be easily pierced with a fork.

STRAWBERRY AND BANANA SMOOTHIE (2 SERVINGS)

Created by Callie

Prep time: 10 minutes

Strawberries and bananas make a delicious combination. This recipe contains a great source of potassium, vitamin C, and calcium and makes a great after school or post-activity drink.

Ingredients:

1. 4 ounces of fresh strawberries

2. 1 banana

3. 4-ounce carton of strawberry probiotic yogurt

4. 4 fluid ounces of milk

Instructions:

Place fruit, yogurt, and milk into a smoothie maker, blender, or food processor and blend until smooth.

BEAN AND TUNA SALAD (4 SERVINGS)

Created by Hallie and her mom

Prep time: 15 minutes

This recipe is rich in protein, B vitamins, iron, and fiber.

Ingredients:

1. 1 tin of cannelloni or butter beans, drained

2. 2 tomatoes (cut in cubes)

3. 1 can of tuna

4. 4-ounce can of green beans, cooked and cooled

5. 1 tablespoon of red wine vinegar

6. 2 tablespoons of olive oil

7. Fresh herbs: chives, parsley

Instructions:

1. Combine the beans, tomatoes, tuna, and green beans into a bowl.

2. Mix together the vinegar, olive oil, and herbs (to taste), and combine with the salad.

GINGERBREAD KIDS

Created by Kim; adapted by Sarah

Prep time: 25 minutes
Cook time: 15 minutes
Bake time: 1 hour, 35 minutes

This recipe is low in fat.

Ingredients:

1. 1 (3.5 ounce) package of cook and serve butterscotch pudding mix

2. ½ cup butter (soften)

3. ½ cup packed brown sugar

4. 1 egg

5. 1 ½ teaspoons ground ginger

6. 1 ½ cups all-purpose flour

7. 1 teaspoon ground cinnamon

8. ½ teaspoon baking soda

Instructions:

1. In a medium bowl, add the dry butterscotch pudding mix, butter, and brown sugar; mix until smooth. Stir in the egg.

2. In another bowl, combine the ginger, flour, baking soda, and cinnamon; combine both mixtures and stir.

3. Cover, and allow dough to chill until firm, approximately one hour.

4. Preheat oven to 350 degrees F.

5. Spray baking sheets with non-stick cooking spray.

6. On a floured board, knead dough with a roller into a uniform mixture to about 1/6-1/8-inch thickness, and use a cookie cutter to cut into man shapes. Place cookies 2-3 inches apart on the baking sheets.

7. Bake in the oven for 10 to 12 minutes or until cookies are golden at the edges.

8. Allow to cool.

9. Optional: decorate with icing.

Thank You

Thank you #FocusBuilders #SuperMoms #ADHDChamps #AllStars for your unwavering support and for purchasing and reading this book. This is the FIRST of many books to come! I would appreciate your feedback and would be grateful if you could take 30 seconds to provide brief remarks on the book's website: www.ADHDLifestyleSeries.com.

I hope you have learned new ways to help your child manage their ADHD symptoms by incorporating healthy meal routines and encouraging age-appropriate activities. With a comprehensive and supportive treatment plan, you will increase your child's likelihood of championing their ADHD so they can function at their optimal level and experience success.

I enjoy what I do. I enjoy helping kids and their families manage their school, social, and home lifestyles while they function with their ADHD. I'm either seeing a patient in one of the three offices I work in, providing consultations to families using a telepsychiatry platform, completing an online, print, radio, or TV media interview, or providing awareness and education about ADHD through my speaker circuit to Moms and their families. I am excited to announce my upcoming LIVE online course that focuses on how to help build your child's All Star ADHD Support Team! Let's stay connected so I can keep you updated on my activities!

Here's how:

WEBSITE:
https://www.DrDawnPsychMD.com

FACEBOOK:
https://www.facebook.com/DrDawnPsychMD

TWITTER:
https://twitter.com/DrDawnPsychMD

YOUTUBE:
https://www.youtube.com/c/DrDawnPsychMD

INSTAGRAM:
https://instagram.com/DrDawnPsychMD

PINTEREST:
https://www.pinterest.com/DrDawnPsychMD

LINKEDIN:
https://www.linkedin.com/in/DrDawnPsychMD

GOOGLE+:
https://www.google.com/+DrDawnPsychMD

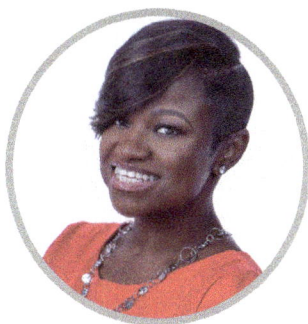

About the Author

Dr. Dawn Brown, "The MD with ADHD," is a double–board certified child, adolescent, and adult psychiatrist. The CEO of ADHD Wellness Center, Dr. Dawn has two private practices in addition to offering online appointments. A nationally recognized pioneer of the Mental Health Movement, Dr. Dawn is on a mission to destigmatize mental illness. She has given over a hundred lectures to residents and child psychiatry fellows, appeared on numerous news and media outlets and helped to establish a health clinic in Houston, Texas.

Originally from Flint, Michigan, Dr. Dawn earned her doctorate degree and completed her residency at the Saint Louis University School of Medicine, and finished an additional two-year fellowship at Baylor College of Medicine. She has been a recurring expert on the nationally syndicated *Tom Joyner Morning Show*, and was awarded Top Psychiatrist by the International Association of Health Care Professionals.

In her spare time, Dr. Dawn enjoys spending time with family and friends, traveling internationally, singing, bowling, and music. She also has two adorable teacup Yorkies.

To connect, visit her website at
www.DrDawnPsychMD.com

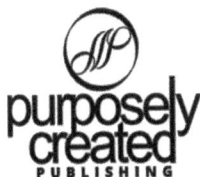

CREATING DISTINCTIVE BOOKS
WITH INTENTIONAL RESULTS

We're a collaborative group of creative masterminds
with a mission to produce high-quality books to position
you for monumental success in the marketplace.

Our professional team of writers, editors, designers,
and marketing strategists work closely together to ensure
that every detail of your book is a clear representation
of the message in your writing.

Want to know more?
Write to us at info@publishyourgift.com
or call (888) 949-6228

Discover great books, exclusive offers, and more at
www.PublishYourGift.com

Connect with us on social media

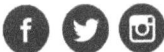

@publishyourgift